DIABETIC FOOT CARE
HANDBOOK & JOURNAL

The Glass Foot

A Plain-English Guide for Patients Living with Diabetes

DR. JAMES WHITFIELD
Reconstructive Foot Surgeon

MELON GLOW BOOKS
Sonoma County, California
www.melonglowbooks.com

Diabetic Foot Care Handbook & Journal

The Glass Foot

Published by Melon Glow Books · Sonoma County, California

www.melonglowbooks.com

ISBN 979-8-9961392-6-2 (Paperback)

ISBN 979-8-9961392-7-9 (Hardcover)

For my patients — every one of whom taught me something.

I have spent nearly thirty years as a foot surgeon. I have operated on feet that were damaged, infected, ulcerated, and broken in every way that feet can be broken. I have sat with patients before surgery and after. I have had the conversations no one wants to have — about what happens when things are caught too late, and about what could have been done differently.

The patients I think about most are not the complicated surgical cases. They are the ones who came in with something small — a blister, a callus, a bit of redness — that had quietly been progressing for weeks because no one had told them what to look for. Because no one had explained, in plain language, what diabetes actually does to a foot, and why that changes everything about how that foot must be cared for.

That is why I wrote this book.

This is not a textbook. It is written for the person sitting at the kitchen table who has just been told they have diabetes and wants to understand what that means for their feet. Plain, direct, and honest about the stakes.

The Glass Foot is the image I always return to. Your foot contains some of the finest, most delicate blood vessels in the body. In a diabetic patient, those vessels are more fragile still. And the foot, being the farthest point from the heart, receives the least of everything the body has to offer.

But here is what I also know after thirty years: most of what goes wrong in a diabetic foot is preventable. The daily inspection. The right shoes. The early treatment of a fungal infection. The habit of shaking out your shoes every morning. These are not complicated things. They are the things that keep small problems from becoming large ones.

The journal section at the back is there for a reason. Use it. Bring it to your appointments. Let it become the record of a foot that is being watched, cared for, and protected every day.

Your feet have been carrying you all your life without asking for much in return. Now they need a little more from you. I hope this book helps you give it to them.

Dr. James Whitfield

Reconstructive Foot Surgeon · Melon Glow Books

CHAPTER ONE

What Boxers Know That Diabetic Patients Don't

The Glass Jaw and the Glass Foot

In boxing, they call it a glass jaw.

One punch in the right spot and the fight is over — no matter how strong, how fast, or how well-trained the fighter is. A glass jaw isn't something you can see from the outside. The fighter looks perfectly healthy. His corner men don't worry. The crowd doesn't notice. But underneath, there is a hidden fragility that one good hit will expose — completely and catastrophically.

Diabetes does the same thing to your feet.

It creates what I call a glass foot — a foot that looks perfectly normal, feels perfectly fine, but can be destroyed by a single small injury you never even noticed.

I spent nearly thirty years as a foot and ankle surgeon. I have stood in operating rooms and removed body parts that could have been saved had the patient come to me sooner. By the time I saw them, the damage had progressed so far that an entire team of specialists — vascular surgeons, infectious disease physicians, wound care nurses — had to be called in, and still we could not always save what should never have been lost. People who felt fine. People who thought they were careful. People who lost everything to a blister they never felt, a cut they never saw, a shoe that fit just a little too tight.

Every one of them had a glass foot. And most of them didn't know it.

HOW DIABETES CREATES THE GLASS FOOT

To understand the glass foot, you need to understand what diabetes quietly does to your feet over time — because it does it without pain, without warning, and without mercy.

It steals your nerve signals.

The medical term is peripheral neuropathy. What it means in plain English is this: the nerves in your feet stop working properly. They stop sending accurate signals to your brain. And the most important signal they stop sending is pain.

Pain is your body's alarm system. It is how you know something is wrong. When you step on a nail, pain tells you instantly. When a shoe rubs a blister, pain tells you to take it off. When a wound is getting infected, pain tells you to see a doctor.

Take away pain, and you take away every warning you have.

THE GLASS JAW vs. THE GLASS FOOT

A boxer with a glass jaw still feels the punch. He goes down, but he knows he's been hit. A diabetic patient with neuropathy may step on a tack, walk on it for three days, and never feel a thing. By the time they notice — if they notice — the wound is already infected.

It cuts off your blood supply.

Diabetes damages blood vessels throughout the body, and the vessels in the feet are among the first to suffer. Poor circulation means that when an injury occurs, the body cannot deliver the oxygen, white blood cells, and nutrients needed to heal it.

On a healthy foot, a small cut heals in days. The body rushes resources to the wound, fights off bacteria, and closes the skin quickly and cleanly.

On a glass foot, that same small cut may not heal for weeks — or ever. The blood simply cannot get there in enough quantity to do the job. Bacteria move in. The infection deepens. It reaches the bone. And at that point, the surgeon's options become very limited.

It makes you unaware of the damage.

Here is what makes the glass foot truly dangerous: the combination of these two problems. No pain to warn you. No circulation to heal you. An injury occurs. You don't feel it. You keep walking on it. The pressure and movement make it worse. The poor blood supply means it cannot heal. Days pass. Weeks pass. By the time it becomes visible — by the time the skin breaks open or the swelling appears or the odor begins — the damage has gone deep.

SURGEON'S NOTE — WHAT I HAVE SEEN

I have seen patients come into my office with wounds they had been walking on for two weeks without knowing it. I have seen bone exposed through wounds that started as blisters. I have seen injuries that, on a healthy foot, would have healed over a weekend — but on a glass foot, required a team of specialists and still ended in permanent loss. This is the glass foot. This is what diabetes does.

THE PUNCH YOU NEVER SEE COMING

A boxer with a glass jaw has one advantage: he knows about it. He trains to protect it. He keeps his guard up. He studies his opponents for the left hook that could end the fight.

Most diabetic patients never get that advantage — because nobody tells them clearly enough what they are dealing with.

They are told their blood sugar is high. They are told to watch their diet. They are given medications. But often, nobody sits them down and says: *Your feet are now made of glass. One wrong step, one ignored blister, one pair of tight shoes — and you could lose something you can never get back.*

I am telling you now.

Your feet require a different level of attention than they did before your diagnosis. Not because they look different. Not because they feel different — in fact, the loss of feeling is precisely the problem. But because the rules have changed. The margin for error that a healthy person has — the ability to ignore a small cut, to wear uncomfortable shoes for one more day, to skip checking their feet before bed — that margin is gone.

You are now handling glass. And glass requires care.

WHAT CAREFUL HANDS LOOK LIKE

When a glassblower works, he does not rush. He does not handle his work carelessly. He inspects it constantly — turning it, examining it from every angle, looking for the tiny flaw that could become a crack, the small imperfection that could spread.

That is what daily foot inspection is. It is the careful hands of someone who knows what they are working with.

THE DAILY INSPECTION — WHAT TO LOOK FOR

Every morning, before you get out of bed, look at your feet. All of them — top, bottom, between the toes, around the nails, at the heel. Use a mirror if you need to. Ask someone to help if you cannot see the bottom. What you are looking for is anything that was not there yesterday: a red spot, a small cut, a blister, a swollen area, skin that looks darker than usual, a nail that is ingrown. These are the small cracks in the glass. Caught early, many of them can be managed. Left alone, any one of them can become the punch that ends the fight.

This handbook exists so that you never get to the point where a team of specialists is required — where reconstructive foot surgery becomes the only option, where amputation enters the conversation. So let's pay attention now, before we ever get to the reconstructive stage.

A SURGEON'S PROMISE

I designed every page of this handbook from the perspective of someone who has seen what happens when the glass foot goes unprotected — and who has also seen what happens when patients take their foot care seriously.

The patients who inspect their feet every day. Who never walk barefoot. Who check their blood sugar consistently. Who bring small concerns to their doctor before they become large ones. Those patients keep their feet. They keep their independence. They keep their lives.

You are holding the tool that can make that difference. Use it every day. Take it seriously. Treat your feet the way you would treat something precious and fragile — because that is exactly what they are.

The glass foot can be protected. But only if you handle it with care.

— Dr. James Whitfield

Foot & Ankle Surgeon, Retired · Nearly 30 years of surgical practice

CHAPTER TWO

The Glass Foot

Why Diabetic Feet Demand Your Full Attention

I want you to picture something. Close your eyes for a moment and imagine that your foot — the one that carries you through every single day — is made entirely of glass. Not thick, sturdy glass, but the finest, most delicate crystal you have ever seen. The kind that rings like a bell when you tap it and shatters at the slightest wrong pressure.

Now imagine walking on that foot. Across the pavement. Across rocks. Into shoes that pinch and rub. Through summer heat and winter cold. Bearing the full weight of your body, step after step, mile after mile, year after year.

THE GLASS FOOT

Imagine your foot is made of glass. The tiny blood vessels — the capillaries and microvasculature — are as fragile as the finest crystal. In a diabetic foot, these vessels are even more delicate, and far harder to repair once damaged.

That image — the glass foot — is the one I want you to carry throughout this handbook. Because for a person living with diabetes, it is not merely a metaphor. It is closer to the truth than most patients ever realize, until it is too late.

THE INVISIBLE DAMAGE INSIDE

Deep inside the foot runs an intricate network of blood vessels. Some are large enough to see. But the ones that matter most in diabetic foot disease are the smallest ones — the capillaries and microvasculature that feed the skin, the nerves, and the tissue at the very edges of circulation. These vessels are extraordinarily fine. They are easily bruised. Easily broken. And in a diabetic patient, they are extraordinarily difficult to repair.

Here is why that matters so much: the foot is the farthest point in your body from your heart. Blood has to travel the longest distance to get there. Pressure is lower. Flow is slower. In a diabetic patient whose circulation is already compromised by years of elevated blood sugar, this becomes a serious medical vulnerability.

SURGEON'S NOTE

In nearly 30 years of foot surgery, I have seen more hospitalizations, amputations, and life-altering complications trace their origin to a small unnoticed wound on the bottom of a foot than from almost any other single cause. A blister. A callus. A pebble in a shoe. These are not small things in a diabetic patient.

THE SILENT THIEF: LOST SENSATION

One of the cruelest complications of long-term diabetes is peripheral neuropathy — the gradual loss of sensation in the feet and lower legs. Your body's normal warning system, the pain that tells you something is wrong, begins to go quiet. A cut doesn't sting the way it should. A developing ulcer on the bottom of the foot may go completely unnoticed for days.

WHEN SMALL PROBLEMS BECOME LIFE-THREATENING

A small ulcer that would heal in days in a healthy person can persist for weeks or months in a diabetic foot. As it lingers, bacteria find their way in. Infection takes hold in tissue that lacks the blood supply to fight back effectively. That local infection can deepen, reaching bone. It can spread. It can become sepsis — a life-threatening whole-body response to infection that sends patients to the hospital, and in the worst cases, to the operating room for an amputation that could have been prevented.

I do not say this to frighten you. I say it because understanding the stakes is the first step toward protecting yourself.

In the chapters ahead, we will walk through exactly how to do that — daily inspections, proper footwear, wound recognition, when to call your doctor, and the simple habits that can make an enormous difference.

CHAPTER THREE

Know Your Enemy

What Diabetes Does to the Foot

The body is a democracy, of sorts. Every organ, every limb, every system makes its demands and draws its share of the body's resources. The brain commands. The heart insists. And the feet — the feet are the quiet ones at the far end of the table, getting along on whatever is left.

> *"The feet are the poor cousins of the body — receiving less nourishment than any other part, yet soldiering on, day after day, without complaint."*

We have already discussed the distance from the heart. And as anyone knows, distance from anything can lead to neglect. Your feet know this. They soldier on regardless — through pavement and gravel, through heat and cold, bearing the full weight of everything you are. But now there is diabetes. And diabetes changes the terms of that arrangement entirely.

A THINNER DINNER PLATE

Think of it this way. Every part of your body sits down each day to a dinner plate — a share of the circulation, the oxygen, the nutrients, the healing resources your body produces. The feet have always had a smaller plate than most. They are at the end of the line.

Diabetes makes that plate thinner still.

Years of elevated blood sugar damage the walls of blood vessels — large ones and small ones alike. The fine capillaries that feed the skin and the nerves of the foot thicken and narrow. Blood flows through them more slowly, in smaller quantities, carrying less of everything the foot needs to stay healthy and repair itself.

SURGEON'S NOTE — THE WHOLE BODY IS AFFECTED

The body is compromised throughout by diabetes — the kidneys, the eyes, the cardiovascular system, the nerves. We are focusing here on the feet, but understand: what diabetes does to the foot, it is doing elsewhere too. The foot is where we see the consequences most vividly — because of where it sits at the very end of the body's supply chain.

THE ENDOCRINE SYSTEM — PLAIN ENGLISH

The endocrine system is the body's chemical messenger network — glands that produce and release hormones directly into the bloodstream. The pancreas produces insulin — the hormone that acts like a key, unlocking cells so they can absorb glucose from the blood. In Type 2 diabetes, the body either does not produce enough insulin, or the cells have become resistant to it — the locks have changed, and the old key no longer fits.

The result: glucose builds up in the bloodstream instead of entering the cells that need it. And that excess glucose quietly damages nerves, stiffens blood vessel walls, impairs the immune system, and reduces the body's capacity to heal.

THE THREE DANGERS

Neuropathy The foot loses its voice	■	Poor Circulation The dinner plate grows thinner	■	Slow Healing Wounds linger and deepen

- **Neuropathy** — nerve damage that silences the foot's alarm system. The foot can be injured and send no signal strong enough to trigger a response.
- **Poor Circulation** — damaged blood vessels mean the foot receives less blood, less oxygen, and fewer resources needed to fight infection

and heal.

• **Slow Healing** — these first two dangers combine to produce the third. A wound that would heal in days in a healthy person may take weeks or months in a diabetic foot.

Your feet have always been the quiet soldiers at the end of the line. Now they need your help — more than ever before — because the plate they are working from has never been thinner.

CHAPTER FOUR

The Daily Foot Inspection

Your Single Most Important Daily Habit

If I could give every diabetic patient one habit — just one — it would be this: look at your feet every single day. Not a glance. A real, deliberate inspection. Because the foot that cannot feel what is happening to it depends entirely on your eyes to catch what its nerves have missed.

This takes two minutes. It costs nothing. And it has prevented more amputations than any surgery I have ever performed.

WHY LOOKING REPLACES FEELING

In a healthy foot, pain is the guardian. It shouts when something is wrong. It stops you mid-step when a pebble enters your shoe. Neuropathy silences that alarm. The injury still happens — the blister, the cut, the developing ulcer — but the signal never reaches you. Your eyes must now do the job your nerves can no longer do reliably.

SURGEON'S NOTE — TWO MINUTES A DAY

I have had patients come in with wounds they had no idea existed. A nail puncture. A blister the size of a quarter. An early ulcer on the heel. Not because they were careless — but because they simply never looked. Two minutes a day changes that entirely.

THE STEP-BY-STEP ROUTINE

- **Top of the foot** — check for redness, swelling, any change in skin color, cuts, or abrasions.
- **Bottom of the foot (sole)** — use a mirror. Look at the heel, the arch, and the ball. These are the highest-pressure areas and the most

common sites for ulcers.

• **Between every toe** — spread the toes gently and look in each space. Fungal infections and skin breakdown often hide here and go undetected longest.

• **The toes and toenails** — check for ingrown nails, bruising, discoloration, or any nail that appears thickened or crumbly.

• **The heel** — feel with your fingers as well as looking. Heel cracks can be deep enough to bleed and become infected without being immediately visible.

• **Skin temperature** — run the back of your hand across both feet. One foot significantly warmer than the other is a warning sign worth investigating.

IMPORTANT — NEVER SKIP THE INSPECTION

If you cannot bend or see your feet clearly, do not skip this inspection. Ask a family member or caregiver to help. Use a long-handled mirror. Consider a podiatry appointment for professional inspection if daily self-inspection is not possible. This step is not optional.

YOUR EYES AND YOUR DOCTOR'S EYES — BOTH MATTER

Daily self-inspection is essential. But your physician's examination is something different entirely. When your doctor examines your feet, he or she is closer to them — physically, professionally, clinically — than you have ever been. The trained eye at that distance sees things a careful patient with a mirror cannot always catch: early tissue changes, subtle color shifts, the beginning of a wound that has not yet broken the surface.

SURGEON'S NOTE — YOUR EYES AND YOUR FEET

The same fragile blood vessels causing problems in your feet are also at work in your eyes. Diabetic retinopathy — bleeding and leakage from tiny vessels in the retina — is one of the leading causes of vision loss in diabetic patients. If your vision is deteriorating — cataracts forming, sight weakening — the very eyes you rely on to inspect your feet may not be giving you a complete picture. See both your foot doctor and your eye doctor regularly. The same disease is at work in both places.

It sneaks up gradually. Do not let any of it sneak up on you. That is the lesson of this entire chapter, and of this entire book.

Your feet have been carrying you in silence for years. Now it is your turn to watch over them — and to bring in the right professional eyes to help. Two minutes every morning. Regular visits to your doctor.

CHAPTER FIVE

Footwear

The Most Underestimated Medicine

In nearly thirty years of foot surgery, I have seen many things send patients to the operating room. But I have also seen something far more preventable cause serious, lasting damage to diabetic feet: the wrong shoes. Or worse — no shoes at all.

SHAKE YOUR SHOES — EVERY SINGLE TIME

Before I say another word about footwear, I want to give you the single most important habit I teach every diabetic patient. It costs nothing. It takes three seconds. And it could save your foot.

Every morning, before you put on your shoes, pick them up and shake them out. Turn them upside down. Look inside. Every single time — not just when you think something might be in there. Because you will not always know.

SURGEON'S TIP — SHAKE YOUR SHOES FIRST

You will be surprised what has been found inside shoes before they were put on. Scorpions. Centipedes. Spiders — and their egg sacs. Bits of gravel or broken glass. A screw. A small pebble. A healthy person feels that foreign object within seconds and removes it. A diabetic patient with neuropathy may feel nothing — and walk on it all day. By the time the skin breaks, an infection is already beginning. Shake your shoes. Every time. No exceptions.

THE INVISIBLE HAZARD — TINY GLASS YOU CANNOT SEE

Think back to the last time a glass broke in your kitchen. You swept up carefully. But glass, when it shatters, does not break into pieces you can always see. The finest fragments are almost dust-like — invisible to the naked eye, light enough to drift, small enough to settle into the gap beneath a dishwasher or along a baseboard.

Then, weeks or months later, a vibration, a breeze, a door closing — and those invisible fragments migrate out onto the floor you walk on every morning. A person with normal sensation feels it immediately and demands it be removed. A diabetic patient who cannot feel it walks on that fragment all day, every step driving it slightly deeper.

A SURGEON'S REFLECTION — ANDROCLES AND THE LION

This situation always reminds me of the fable of Androcles and the Lion. Androcles encounters a lion roaring in agony in a cave. He bravely removes a large thorn buried deep in the lion's paw and cleans the wound. They part as friends. Later, Androcles is thrown into the arena to be devoured by a lion — the same one. It recognizes him, refuses to attack, and shows him only affection. The emperor, moved, frees them both. A thorn in a paw. A sliver of glass in a foot. The principle is the same: a small foreign body, left unaddressed, causes constant suffering. Removed with skill and care — it changes everything.

WHAT TO LOOK FOR IN DIABETIC-SAFE FOOTWEAR

- **Deep toe box** — enough room for all five toes to lie flat without compression.
- **Cushioned sole** — thick enough to absorb impact and protect from hard surfaces.
- **Smooth interior lining** — no prominent seams or rough stitching against the skin.
- **Adjustable closure** — laces or velcro allow you to customize fit as swelling changes through the day.

- **Breathable material** — moisture trapped inside a shoe invites fungal infection.
- **Proper length** — half an inch of space between the longest toe and the end of the shoe.

IMPORTANT — DO NOT 'BREAK IN' SHOES

Never buy shoes that feel tight and expect them to 'break in.' A diabetic foot cannot afford that process. Buy shoes that fit correctly from day one.

NEVER GO BAREFOOT — THE SURGEON'S FIRM RULE

Never walk barefoot. Not in your house. Not on the beach. Not on the grass. Not from the bed to the bathroom at 2 in the morning. I have treated patients who stepped on a staple in their own living room and did not feel it. I have treated patients who burned the soles of their feet on hot pavement at the beach and did not realize it until they saw the blisters.

Keep a pair of clean, well-fitting slippers next to your bed. Put them on before your feet touch the floor. This is not excessive caution. This is simply understanding what your foot can and cannot feel — and protecting it accordingly.

The right shoes, the right socks, the habit of shaking them out every morning, and never letting bare skin touch an unprotected floor — these carry enormous protective power for a diabetic foot.

CHAPTER SIX

Skin & Nail Care

The Details That Save Lives

We have already talked at length about the poor circulation that defines the diabetic foot — the fine, fragile vessels, the slow healing, the daily trauma of simply walking through life. Given everything we know about how the diabetic foot functions — warm, poorly circulated, often damp inside a shoe for hours at a time — it should come as no surprise that this is an excellent breeding ground for fungal infection.

FUNGAL INFECTIONS — THE QUIET THREAT THAT ESCALATES FAST

Fungi thrive in warm, moist, low-circulation environments. The diabetic foot provides exactly those conditions. Left untreated, a fungal infection softens, cracks, and breaks down the skin barrier — the body's first line of defense against bacteria. Once that barrier is breached, what began as a patch of athlete's foot can progress to a skin ulceration, then to a deeper infection, with serious consequences.

Poor Circu lation	■	Warm & Moist Foot	■	Fungal Infection	■	Skin Brea kdown	■	Ulceration

This chain is entirely preventable — but only if the fungal infection is caught and treated on time. At the first sign of infection, before the skin has been compromised.

SURGEON'S TIP — RECOGNIZE FUNGAL INFECTION EARLY

Look for: skin that appears white, soggy, or peeling between the toes. Redness, scaling, or flaking on the sole or sides of the foot. Thickened, discolored, or crumbly toenails. Any persistent itching — though many diabetic patients feel none at all. If you see any of these signs, do not wait. Treat immediately or call your doctor.

MOISTURIZING — WHAT TO USE, AND WHERE NOT TO APPLY IT

Dry, cracked skin is another entry point for infection. Poor circulation means the diabetic foot often produces less natural oil, leading to dryness — particularly on the heel, which bears tremendous daily pressure.

Moisturize your feet daily after bathing, while the skin is still slightly damp. Use a fragrance-free lotion or cream — urea-based creams (10–25%) are particularly effective for thickened or very dry skin.

IMPORTANT — NEVER MOISTURIZE BETWEEN THE TOES

Do NOT apply moisturizer between the toes. Moisture trapped in those spaces promotes exactly the warm, damp environment that fungal infections need to take hold. Between the toes stays dry.

NAIL CARE — STRAIGHT ACROSS, NEVER TOO SHORT

- **Cut straight across** — never curve the corners down into the nail groove.
- **Leave a small white margin** — do not cut so short that the nail no longer extends past the skin edge.
- **Use proper nail scissors or clippers** — clean, sharp instruments only. Dull clippers tear rather than cut.
- **File sharp edges** — use an emery board to smooth any rough corners after cutting.

- **If you cannot see or reach your feet safely** — see a podiatrist regularly for nail care.

The skin is the foot's armor. In a diabetic patient, that armor is thinner, slower to repair, and surrounded by conditions that favor its enemies. Keep it intact through daily moisturizing, early treatment of fungal infections, and careful nail care.

CHAPTER SEVEN

Red Flags

When to Call Your Doctor Immediately

Everything we have discussed in this book is aimed at prevention. But prevention is not a guarantee. When wounds develop, the single most important thing a diabetic patient can do is recognize the warning signs early and act without delay.

Time is not neutral in a diabetic foot wound. Every day of delay is a day the infection has to deepen, to spread, to establish itself in tissue that cannot fight back effectively. What is treatable on Monday with antibiotics and wound care may require surgery by Friday.

THE FIRST RULE — DO NOT WAIT

If you see any of the signs listed in this chapter — do not wait. Do not watch it for a few more days. Do not assume it will resolve on its own. Call your doctor the same day. If after hours, go to urgent care. If there is fever, spreading redness, or you feel systemically unwell — go to the ER.

WARNING SIGNS NO DIABETIC PATIENT SHOULD IGNORE

- Any wound that has not begun to improve within 24–48 hours of basic home care
- Redness spreading beyond the immediate edge of a wound
- Warmth, swelling, or tenderness in or around any wound
- Any discharge from a wound — clear, cloudy, or discolored
- A wound with an odor — a serious sign of bacterial activity
- Skin that appears dark, dusky, or black around a wound
- Fever, chills, or feeling generally unwell alongside any foot wound

• Any wound on the foot that you did not notice forming

ULCERS, INFECTION, AND THE ROAD TO AMPUTATION

A diabetic foot ulcer is an open wound — a breakdown of the skin that exposes the tissue beneath. Ulcers are often painless in patients with neuropathy, which is precisely what makes them so dangerous. Left untreated, the wound deepens, bacteria colonize it, infection spreads into surrounding tissue (cellulitis), and from there can reach the bone itself (osteomyelitis). Bone infections are extremely difficult to treat and often require surgical removal of infected bone tissue.

SURGEON'S NOTE — THE ROAD TO AMPUTATION

The road to amputation is not sudden. It is a series of missed opportunities — each one small, each one manageable, if caught and treated at the right time. A blister becomes an ulcer. An ulcer becomes infected. An infection reaches bone. Bone infection leads to the operating room. Every step of that chain can be interrupted. But only if the patient acts early.

YOU ARE AT THE CENTER OF A TEAM

By now you are beginning to realize something important: the feet we have been focusing on throughout this book are part of a whole. If you are living with diabetes, you have probably already met the team of specialists that whole person requires.

• **Your internist** — the quarterback of your overall medical care, tracking the whole picture

• **Your endocrinologist** — managing your blood sugar and the underlying diabetic condition

• **Your ophthalmologist** — watching the fragile vessels of the retina for early damage

- **Your foot surgeon or podiatrist** — protecting and treating the feet
- **And in rural areas** — the good old family doctor, quietly quarterbacking the whole effort

SURGEON'S NOTE — YOUR WHOLE TEAM IS WATCHING

No single specialist sees all of you. That is why the team exists. Be a cooperative patient. Keep your appointments with all of them. Bring your journal. Tell each one what the others have said. You are not just a foot, or an eye, or a blood sugar number. You are a whole person — and your whole team knows it.

There is no small wound in a diabetic foot. There is only a wound that has been caught early — or one that has not. The chapters you have read, and the team of professionals watching over you, give you everything you need.

BONUS CHAPTER

Gout

When the Big Toe Roars

As a foot surgeon, gout is one of the most common conditions I treat — and one of the most dramatic. When gout strikes, there is no mistaking it. Patients describe it as the worst pain they have ever felt. Grown men who have survived broken bones and major surgery tell me a gout attack brought them to their knees. The bedsheet touching the toe is agony. The air in the room feels like too much.

WHAT GOUT ACTUALLY IS

Gout is a form of inflammatory arthritis caused by the buildup of uric acid in the blood. When uric acid levels climb too high, the excess crystallizes — forming tiny, needle-sharp crystals that deposit in the joints and surrounding tissue. The big toe joint is the most common target, though the ankle, heel, and knee can all be affected.

SURGEON'S NOTE — YOU WILL KNOW WHEN IT IS GOUT

Gout attacks often strike at night — waking patients from sleep with sudden, severe pain in the big toe joint. If you have never had gout, you will know immediately when you do. Either way — call your doctor. Do not wait it out.

WHY DIABETIC PATIENTS ARE AT HIGHER RISK

High blood sugar. Insulin resistance. Excess weight. A diet heavy in red meat, organ meats, shellfish, and alcohol. All of these raise uric acid levels. All of these are also primary drivers of Type 2 diabetes. The patient who arrives in my office with a gout attack very often has a blood chemistry panel that tells a much larger story.

> *"High blood sugar, insulin resistance, and a diet of excess leads to a blood chemistry that is, to put it mildly, outrageous — and the kidneys are the ones paying the price."*

THE KIDNEYS — THE ORGAN YOU FORGOT ABOUT

Uric acid is processed and excreted by the kidneys. When the kidneys are working well, they filter uric acid efficiently. But diabetes damages the kidneys — quietly, gradually, over years of elevated blood sugar. When the kidneys are compromised, they cannot clear uric acid as effectively. Levels build up in the blood. Crystals form. Gout follows.

IMPORTANT — GOUT IS A WHOLE-BODY WARNING SIGN

Elevated uric acid in a diabetic patient is not just a gout problem. It is a signal that the kidneys may be under stress. Your internist and endocrinologist need to know about every gout attack. Blood chemistry — uric acid, creatinine, kidney function — must be monitored regularly.

A CONVERSATION WORTH HAVING

When a patient comes in with gout — especially a diabetic patient whose blood panel tells the whole story — there is a conversation that needs to happen. Not just about the toe. About everything.

THE COUNTRY DOCTOR'S CONVERSATION

The good country doctor — the family physician who knows you and your family — has a particular gift for this moment. He will look at your chart, your blood work, and you, and put it all together. And he may well say: I want someone else in the room for this conversation. A spouse. A son or daughter. Someone who will help you listen. Because what he has to tell you is important. The blood sugar. The uric acid. The kidney numbers. The weight. The direction things are heading — and where they can go if nothing changes. That is not a conversation meant to frighten you. It is a conversation meant to save you.

WHAT TO DO WHEN GOUT STRIKES

- **Call your doctor the same day** — anti-inflammatory medications work best when started early
- **Rest the foot** — keep weight off the affected joint as much as possible
- **Elevate** — raise the foot above heart level to help reduce swelling
- **Stay hydrated** — drink plenty of water to help the kidneys flush uric acid
- **Do not self-medicate with aspirin** — aspirin can actually raise uric acid levels and worsen an attack
- **Follow up on blood chemistry** — after the attack resolves, work with your team on long-term uric acid management

Gout announces itself loudly enough that even the most reluctant patient picks up the phone. Use that moment. Call your doctor. Get the full picture. Let your team put it all together for you. That is what they are there for.

How to Use This Section

The journal pages that follow are your daily record of foot health. They are designed to take no more than two to three minutes to complete — the same two minutes you are already spending on your daily inspection.

Consistency is everything. A journal filled out six days out of seven for six months is far more valuable — to you and to your doctor — than a perfect record kept for two weeks and then abandoned.

HOW TO USE EACH DAILY LOG PAGE

- **Date & Day** — fill in at the top so your record stays in order.
- **Inspection Checklist** — check each area you examined. Circle if you found something and note it in the observations box.
- **Pain or Discomfort** — even if sensation is reduced, note any unusual feelings. Rate 0–10.
- **Skin & Nail Notes** — any changes in moisture, cracking, fungal signs, or nail appearance.
- **Footwear** — note what shoes you wore today.
- **Observations** — free space for anything you noticed. A small mark. A color change. A question for your doctor.
- **Action Taken** — note if you applied cream, treated an area, or called your doctor.

BRINGING THIS JOURNAL TO YOUR APPOINTMENTS

Bring this journal to every podiatry or physician appointment. It gives your doctor a window into what has been happening between visits — far more useful than trying to remember weeks of history on the spot. Your doctor can review trends, catch patterns, and adjust your care plan accordingly.

DAILY FOOT CARE LOG **Day 1**

DATE: ______________________ **DAY:** ________________

INSPECTION CHECKLIST (circle any area where you found an issue)

Top of foot (L)	Top of foot (R)	Sole / heel (L)
Sole / heel (R)	Between toes (L)	Between toes (R)
Toenails (L)	Toenails (R)	Skin temperature

OBSERVATIONS

____

____

____

PAIN / DISCOMFORT (0 = none 10 = severe) **0 1 2 3 4 5 6 7 8 9 10**	**FOOTWEAR WORN TODAY** ____________________

SKIN & NAIL NOTES ____________________ ____________________	**ACTION TAKEN** ____________________ ____________________

FUNGAL / INFECTION SIGNS:

■ Peeling between toes ■ Scaling on sole ■ Discolored nail

■ Odor present ■ Redness / warmth ■ None observed

NOTES / QUESTIONS FOR DOCTOR

____

____

____

Diabetic Foot Care Handbook & Journal · Dr. James Whitfield · Melon Glow Books

DAILY FOOT CARE LOG — Day 2

DATE: ____________________ **DAY:** ______________

INSPECTION CHECKLIST (circle any area where you found an issue)

Top of foot (L)	Top of foot (R)	Sole / heel (L)
Sole / heel (R)	Between toes (L)	Between toes (R)
Toenails (L)	Toenails (R)	Skin temperature

OBSERVATIONS

____

____

____

PAIN / DISCOMFORT (0 = none 10 = severe)	FOOTWEAR WORN TODAY
0 1 2 3 4 5 6 7 8 9 10	______________________

SKIN & NAIL NOTES	ACTION TAKEN
______________________	______________________
______________________	______________________

FUNGAL / INFECTION SIGNS:

- ■ Peeling between toes
- ■ Scaling on sole
- ■ Discolored nail
- ■ Odor present
- ■ Redness / warmth
- ■ None observed

NOTES / QUESTIONS FOR DOCTOR

____

____

____

Diabetic Foot Care Handbook & Journal · Dr. James Whitfield · Melon Glow Books

DAILY FOOT CARE LOG — Day 3

DATE: ______________________ DAY: ________________

INSPECTION CHECKLIST (circle any area where you found an issue)

Top of foot (L)	Top of foot (R)	Sole / heel (L)
Sole / heel (R)	Between toes (L)	Between toes (R)
Toenails (L)	Toenails (R)	Skin temperature

OBSERVATIONS

____

____

____

PAIN / DISCOMFORT (0 = none 10 = severe)	FOOTWEAR WORN TODAY
0 1 2 3 4 5 6 7 8 9 10	______________________

SKIN & NAIL NOTES	ACTION TAKEN
______________________	______________________
______________________	______________________

FUNGAL / INFECTION SIGNS:

- ■ Peeling between toes
- ■ Scaling on sole
- ■ Discolored nail
- ■ Odor present
- ■ Redness / warmth
- ■ None observed

NOTES / QUESTIONS FOR DOCTOR

____

____

____

Diabetic Foot Care Handbook & Journal · Dr. James Whitfield · Melon Glow Books

DAILY FOOT CARE LOG **Day 4**

DATE: ______________________ **DAY:** ________________

INSPECTION CHECKLIST (circle any area where you found an issue)

Top of foot (L)	Top of foot (R)	Sole / heel (L)
Sole / heel (R)	Between toes (L)	Between toes (R)
Toenails (L)	Toenails (R)	Skin temperature

OBSERVATIONS

PAIN / DISCOMFORT (0 = none 10 = severe)

0 1 2 3 4 5 6 7 8 9 10

FOOTWEAR WORN TODAY

SKIN & NAIL NOTES

ACTION TAKEN

FUNGAL / INFECTION SIGNS:

- ■ Peeling between toes
- ■ Scaling on sole
- ■ Discolored nail
- ■ Odor present
- ■ Redness / warmth
- ■ None observed

NOTES / QUESTIONS FOR DOCTOR

Diabetic Foot Care Handbook & Journal · Dr. James Whitfield · Melon Glow Books

DAILY FOOT CARE LOG Day 5

DATE: ____________ DAY: ____________

INSPECTION CHECKLIST (circle any area where you found an issue)

Top of foot (L)	Top of foot (R)	Sole / heel (L)
Sole / heel (R)	Between toes (L)	Between toes (R)
Toenails (L)	Toenails (R)	Skin temperature

OBSERVATIONS

PAIN / DISCOMFORT (0 = none 10 = severe) **0 1 2 3 4 5 6 7 8 9 10**	**FOOTWEAR WORN TODAY**
SKIN & NAIL NOTES	**ACTION TAKEN**

FUNGAL / INFECTION SIGNS:

- ■ Peeling between toes
- ■ Scaling on sole
- ■ Discolored nail
- ■ Odor present
- ■ Redness / warmth
- ■ None observed

NOTES / QUESTIONS FOR DOCTOR

Diabetic Foot Care Handbook & Journal · Dr. James Whitfield · Melon Glow Books

DAILY FOOT CARE LOG Day 6

DATE: ____________________ **DAY:** ______________

INSPECTION CHECKLIST (circle any area where you found an issue)

Top of foot (L)	Top of foot (R)	Sole / heel (L)
Sole / heel (R)	Between toes (L)	Between toes (R)
Toenails (L)	Toenails (R)	Skin temperature

OBSERVATIONS

PAIN / DISCOMFORT (0 = none 10 = severe)

0 1 2 3 4 5 6 7 8 9 10

FOOTWEAR WORN TODAY

SKIN & NAIL NOTES

ACTION TAKEN

FUNGAL / INFECTION SIGNS:

- ■ Peeling between toes
- ■ Scaling on sole
- ■ Discolored nail
- ■ Odor present
- ■ Redness / warmth
- ■ None observed

NOTES / QUESTIONS FOR DOCTOR

Diabetic Foot Care Handbook & Journal · Dr. James Whitfield · Melon Glow Books

DAILY FOOT CARE LOG — Day 7

DATE: ____________ DAY: ____________

INSPECTION CHECKLIST (circle any area where you found an issue)

Top of foot (L)	Top of foot (R)	Sole / heel (L)
Sole / heel (R)	Between toes (L)	Between toes (R)
Toenails (L)	Toenails (R)	Skin temperature

OBSERVATIONS

PAIN / DISCOMFORT (0 = none 10 = severe)

0 1 2 3 4 5 6 7 8 9 10

FOOTWEAR WORN TODAY

SKIN & NAIL NOTES

ACTION TAKEN

FUNGAL / INFECTION SIGNS:

- ■ Peeling between toes
- ■ Scaling on sole
- ■ Discolored nail
- ■ Odor present
- ■ Redness / warmth
- ■ None observed

NOTES / QUESTIONS FOR DOCTOR

Diabetic Foot Care Handbook & Journal · Dr. James Whitfield · Melon Glow Books

WEEKLY SUMMARY & DOCTOR'S NOTES

WEEK OF: ____________________________

OVERALL ASSESSMENT THIS WEEK:

- ■ No issues — feet in good condition
- ■ Minor issue identified and treated
- ■ Issue present — monitoring closely
- ■ Called / saw doctor this week

ISSUES OR CONCERNS THIS WEEK:

TREATMENTS OR ACTIONS TAKEN:

QUESTIONS TO ASK MY DOCTOR AT NEXT VISIT:

DOCTOR'S NOTES / APPOINTMENT SUMMARY:

Diabetic Foot Care Handbook & Journal · Dr. James Whitfield · Melon Glow Books

WEEKLY SUMMARY & DOCTOR'S NOTES

WEEK OF: ______________________________

OVERALL ASSESSMENT THIS WEEK:

- ■ No issues — feet in good condition
- ■ Minor issue identified and treated
- ■ Issue present — monitoring closely
- ■ Called / saw doctor this week

ISSUES OR CONCERNS THIS WEEK:

TREATMENTS OR ACTIONS TAKEN:

QUESTIONS TO ASK MY DOCTOR AT NEXT VISIT:

DOCTOR'S NOTES / APPOINTMENT SUMMARY:

Diabetic Foot Care Handbook & Journal · Dr. James Whitfield · Melon Glow Books

MEDICATION LOG

A Complete Record for Your Entire Care Team

Your medications are a critical part of managing diabetes and protecting your feet. This log is designed to be brought to every appointment so your entire care team can see at a glance what you are taking, at what dose, and for how long. Never stop or change a medication without consulting your physician. Note any side effects you observe, particularly any that affect your feet or legs.

MEDICATION LOG

List all medications — prescription, over-the-counter, and supplements. Bring this log to every appointment

Medication Name	Dose	Frequency	Prescribing Doctor	Start Date	Notes / Side Effects
1					
2					
3					
4					
5					
6					
7					
8					
9					
10					
11					
12					
13					
14					

KNOWN ALLERGIES / DRUG REACTIONS:

MEDICATION LOG

List all medications — prescription, over-the-counter, and supplements. Bring this log to every appointment.

Medication Name	Dose	Frequency	Prescribing Doctor	Start Date	Notes / Side Effects
15					
16					
17					
18					
19					
20					
21					
22					
23					
24					
25					
26					
27					
28					

KNOWN ALLERGIES / DRUG REACTIONS:

BLOOD SUGAR LOG

Daily Glucose Tracking — Fasting & Post-Meal

Blood sugar management is the foundation of diabetic foot protection. Elevated glucose damages the blood vessels and nerves that your feet depend on. This log tracks your fasting reading — taken before eating in the morning — and your post-meal reading, taken two hours after a meal. Your target ranges will be set by your physician, but in general: fasting below 130 mg/dL and post-meal below 180 mg/dL are commonly recommended starting points. Consistent logging over 60 days gives your doctor a far clearer picture than a single office reading ever can.

BLOOD SUGAR LOG

TARGET RANGES (confirm with doctor): Fasting: under 130 mg/dL | Post-Meal (2 hrs): under 180 mg/dL | Mar

Day	Date	Fasting (mg/dL)	Post-Meal (mg/dL)	Time Taken	Notes / How Feeling
1					
2					
3					
4					
5					
6					
7					
8					
9					
10					
11					
12					
13					
14					
15					

BLOOD SUGAR LOG

TARGET RANGES (confirm with doctor): Fasting: under 130 mg/dL | Post-Meal (2 hrs): under 180 mg/dL

Day	Date	Fasting (mg/dL)	Post-Meal (mg/dL)	Time Taken	Notes / How Feeling
16					
17					
18					
19					
20					
21					
22					
23					
24					
25					
26					
27					
28					
29					
30					

BLOOD SUGAR LOG

TARGET RANGES (confirm with doctor): Fasting: under 130 mg/dL | Post-Meal (2 hrs): under 180 mg/dL | Mark

Day	Date	Fasting (mg/dL)	Post-Meal (mg/dL)	Time Taken	Notes / How Feeling
31					
32					
33					
34					
35					
36					
37					
38					
39					
40					
41					
42					
43					
44					
45					

BLOOD SUGAR LOG

TARGET RANGES (confirm with doctor): Fasting: under 130 mg/dL | Post-Meal (2 hrs): under 180 mg/d

Day	Date	Fasting (mg/dL)	Post-Meal (mg/dL)	Time Taken	Notes / How Feeling
46					
47					
48					
49					
50					
51					
52					
53					
54					
55					
56					
57					
58					
59					
60					

WOUND & INCIDENT LOG

A Permanent Record of Every Skin Event

In a diabetic foot, there is no such thing as a wound too small to document. This log creates a permanent record of every cut, blister, abrasion, redness, or skin change you notice — when it appeared, where it was located, what you did, and how it resolved. Over time, this record reveals patterns your doctor can use to identify problems before they become serious. When in doubt, document it.

WOUND & INCIDENT LOG

Document every skin change, cut, blister, redness, or wound — no matter how minor it appears.

INCIDENT #1

Date noticed: ______ **Left / Right foot:** ______

Location on foot: ______

Description:

______

______

Action taken: ______ **Outcome:** ______

Called doctor? ■ Yes ■ No **Instructions:** ______

INCIDENT #2

Date noticed: ______ **Left / Right foot:** ______

Location on foot: ______

Description:

______

______

Action taken: ______ **Outcome:** ______

Called doctor? ■ Yes ■ No **Instructions:** ______

INCIDENT #3

Date noticed: ______ **Left / Right foot:** ______

Location on foot: ______

Description:

______

______

Action taken: ______ **Outcome:** ______

Called doctor? ■ Yes ■ No **Instructions:** ______

INCIDENT #4

Date noticed: ______ **Left / Right foot:** ______

Location on foot: ______

Description:

______

______

Action taken: ______ **Outcome:** ______

Called doctor? ■ Yes ■ No **Instructions:** ______

WOUND & INCIDENT LOG

Document every skin change, cut, blister, redness, or wound — no matter how minor it appears.

INCIDENT #5

Date noticed: **Left / Right foot:**

Location on foot:

Description:

Action taken: **Outcome:**

Called doctor? ■ **Yes** ■ **No** **Instructions:**

INCIDENT #6

Date noticed: **Left / Right foot:**

Location on foot:

Description:

Action taken: **Outcome:**

Called doctor? ■ **Yes** ■ **No** **Instructions:**

INCIDENT #7

Date noticed: **Left / Right foot:**

Location on foot:

Description:

Action taken: **Outcome:**

Called doctor? ■ **Yes** ■ **No** **Instructions:**

INCIDENT #8

Date noticed: **Left / Right foot:**

Location on foot:

Description:

Action taken: **Outcome:**

Called doctor? ■ **Yes** ■ **No** **Instructions:**

MY CARE TEAM

Every Specialist. Every Number. In One Place.

Bring this page to every appointment. When one specialist asks who else you are seeing, you will have the answer at your fingertips.

Primary Care / Internist

The quarterback of your overall medical care

Name: ______________________ Phone: ______________________

Endocrinologist

Manages your diabetes, blood sugar, and insulin

Name: ______________________ Phone: ______________________

Foot Surgeon / Podiatrist

Protects and treats your feet

Name: ______________________ Phone: ______________________

Ophthalmologist / Eye Doctor

Monitors diabetic changes in the retina

Name: ______________________ Phone: ______________________

Cardiologist

Monitors cardiovascular health

Name: ______________________ Phone: ______________________

Vascular Surgeon

Evaluates blood flow to the legs and feet

Name: ______________________ Phone: ______________________

Wound Care Specialist

Manages chronic or complex wounds

Name: ______________________ Phone: ______________________

Pharmacist

Reviews medications and interactions

Name: ______________________ Phone: ______________________

UPCOMING APPOINTMENTS

Write your questions down before each appointment — you will remember more and your doctor will appreciate it.

1

Date & Time: **Doctor:**

Purpose:

Questions:

2

Date & Time: **Doctor:**

Purpose:

Questions:

3

Date & Time: **Doctor:**

Purpose:

Questions:

4

Date & Time: **Doctor:**

Purpose:

Questions:

5

Date & Time: **Doctor:**

Purpose:

Questions:

6

Date & Time: **Doctor:**

Purpose:

Questions:

7

Date & Time: **Doctor:**

Purpose:

Questions:

APPOINTMENT SUMMARY

Date of appointment: ______________________

Doctor / Specialist seen: ______________________

Location / Clinic: ______________________

Reason for visit: ______________________

WHAT THE DOCTOR FOUND

CHANGES TO MEDICATIONS OR TREATMENT

INSTRUCTIONS GIVEN

FOLLOW-UP REQUIRED

MY NOTES & QUESTIONS FOR NEXT TIME

APPOINTMENT SUMMARY

Date of appointment: ____________________

Doctor / Specialist seen: ____________________

Location / Clinic: ____________________

Reason for visit: ____________________

WHAT THE DOCTOR FOUND

CHANGES TO MEDICATIONS OR TREATMENT

INSTRUCTIONS GIVEN

FOLLOW-UP REQUIRED

MY NOTES & QUESTIONS FOR NEXT TIME

UNDERSTANDING YOUR A1C

The Single Most Important Number in Diabetic Foot Health

A plain-English explanation from Dr. James Whitfield

If you have diabetes, you have probably had your A1C tested. But many patients leave the office without a clear understanding of what that number actually means — and why it matters so profoundly for the health of their feet.

WHAT THE A1C MEASURES

The A1C test measures your average blood sugar level over the past two to three months — not just what it was this morning, but the cumulative picture. It measures how much glucose has attached to the hemoglobin in your red blood cells. A higher A1C means higher average blood sugar over that period.

A1C Level	What It Means	Avg Blood Sugar
Below 5.7%	Normal	Below 117 mg/dL
5.7% – 6.4%	Pre-diabetes	117–137 mg/dL
6.5% and above	Diabetes	137+ mg/dL
Below 7.0%	Well-managed (target)	Below 154 mg/dL
7.0% – 8.0%	Moderate — room to improve	154–183 mg/dL
Above 8.0%	**Elevated risk — feet in danger**	Above 183 mg/dL

WHY THIS MATTERS FOR YOUR FEET: Every point your A1C rises above 7.0% represents meaningful additional damage to the blood vessels and nerves that protect your feet. The goal of this journal is to give you and your doctor the tools to keep that number where it needs to be.

Ask your doctor what your personal A1C target is, and write it here: ___________ Ask how often it should be tested: ___________

SHOE & INSOLE RECORD

Track What You Wear — Your Feet Depend On It

The shoes you wear are the single most controllable risk factor in diabetic foot protection. This record helps you track each pair — when you bought them, any problems they caused, and when they need replacing. A good diabetic shoe typically needs replacement every 6–12 months. Never wear a shoe that caused a blister or skin irritation without having it assessed.

SHOE / INSOLE #1

Brand / Model: ______ **Size:** ______ **Date purchased:** ______

Type: ■ Everyday ■ Diabetic/Therapeutic ■ Athletic ■ Dress ■ Slipper ■ Insole only

Fit notes / problems: ______ ■ In use ■ Retired

SHOE / INSOLE #2

Brand / Model: ______ **Size:** ______ **Date purchased:** ______

Type: ■ Everyday ■ Diabetic/Therapeutic ■ Athletic ■ Dress ■ Slipper ■ Insole only

Fit notes / problems: ______ ■ In use ■ Retired

SHOE / INSOLE #3

Brand / Model: ______ **Size:** ______ **Date purchased:** ______

Type: ■ Everyday ■ Diabetic/Therapeutic ■ Athletic ■ Dress ■ Slipper ■ Insole only

Fit notes / problems: ______ ■ In use ■ Retired

SHOE / INSOLE #4

Brand / Model: ______ **Size:** ______ **Date purchased:** ______

Type: ■ Everyday ■ Diabetic/Therapeutic ■ Athletic ■ Dress ■ Slipper ■ Insole only

Fit notes / problems: ______ ■ In use ■ Retired

SHOE / INSOLE #5

Brand / Model: ______ **Size:** ______ **Date purchased:** ______

Type: ■ Everyday ■ Diabetic/Therapeutic ■ Athletic ■ Dress ■ Slipper ■ Insole only

Fit notes / problems: ______ ■ In use ■ Retired

SHOE / INSOLE #6

Brand / Model: ______ **Size:** ______ **Date purchased:** ______

Type: ■ Everyday ■ Diabetic/Therapeutic ■ Athletic ■ Dress ■ Slipper ■ Insole only

Fit notes / problems: ______ ■ In use ■ Retired

QUICK REFERENCE

Daily Diabetic Foot Care At a Glance

EVERY MORNING

✓ Shake out both shoes and look inside before putting them on

✓ Put on clean, seamless, moisture-wicking socks

✓ Slippers first — never bare feet on the floor

DAILY FOOT INSPECTION

✓ Top of both feet — color, swelling, any new marks

✓ Bottom (sole) — use a mirror; check heel, arch, ball

✓ Between every toe — spread and look carefully

✓ Toenails — discoloration, thickness, ingrown edges

✓ Temperature — one warmer foot is a warning sign

SKIN & NAIL CARE

✓ Moisturize daily after bathing — NOT between the toes

✓ Cut toenails straight across, never too short

✓ Treat any fungal signs immediately — do not wait

✓ No razor blades or chemical corn removers

CALL YOUR DOCTOR TODAY IF:

• Any wound not improving within 24–48 hours • Redness or swelling spreading outward from a wound • Any discharge, odor, or darkening of tissue • Fever or feeling unwell alongside any foot wound • Any wound you did not feel forming

THE SURGEON'S FIRM RULES

• Never go barefoot — not even across the room • Never buy tight shoes expecting to break them in • Never ignore a small wound — there is no small wound here • Never delay calling your doctor when a red flag appears

---

Melon Glow Books · Dr. James Whitfield · www.melonglowbooks.com

Dr. James Whitfield

Reconstructive Foot Surgeon

Dr. James Whitfield is a reconstructive foot surgeon with nearly thirty years of clinical practice, licensed across multiple states. Over the course of his career he has treated thousands of patients suffering from conditions ranging from acute foot injuries to the complex, chronic complications of diabetic foot disease.

His approach to patient care has always been grounded in plain-language education — the belief that patients who understand what is happening in their bodies make better decisions and achieve better outcomes. It is this philosophy that led him to write the Diabetic Foot Care Handbook & Journal.

His clinical experience encompasses reconstructive foot surgery, diabetic wound care, limb salvage, and the surgical management of foot and ankle disorders. He has seen firsthand the difference that early education and daily vigilance make in the lives of diabetic patients — and the devastating consequences when that knowledge is absent.

Dr. Whitfield publishes under the Melon Glow Books imprint, an independent publishing house dedicated to bringing expert medical knowledge to everyday readers in accessible, beautifully crafted books.

Melon Glow Books · Sonoma County, California

ALSO FROM DR. JAMES WHITFIELD

If you have read this far, you already know something important: diabetes does not affect the foot in isolation. It changes the entire environment in which your feet must live and function.

And there is another category of foot conditions that diabetic patients face at higher rates, with more serious consequences — the mechanical and inflammatory conditions that create exactly the kind of pressure, friction, and tissue stress that a diabetic foot can least afford.

Plantar fasciitis. Bone spurs. Arthritis. Gout. The next book in this series was written for you.

COMING NEXT FROM MELON GLOW BOOKS

Plantar Fasciitis, Bone Spurs, Arthritis and Gout

Oh My!

A Plain English Guide for Diabetic Patients

Dr. James Whitfield

In the same plain-English style as this handbook, Dr. Whitfield walks you through each of these conditions — what causes them, what they feel like, and what can be done about them. With special attention throughout to the diabetic patient.

Watch for it at melonglowbooks.com and wherever books are sold.

www.melonglowbooks.com · Support@melonglowbooks.com

www.ingramcontent.com/pod-product-compliance
Lightning Source LLC
LaVergne TN
LVHW010055220926
848484LV00005BA/1218